Mental Fitness

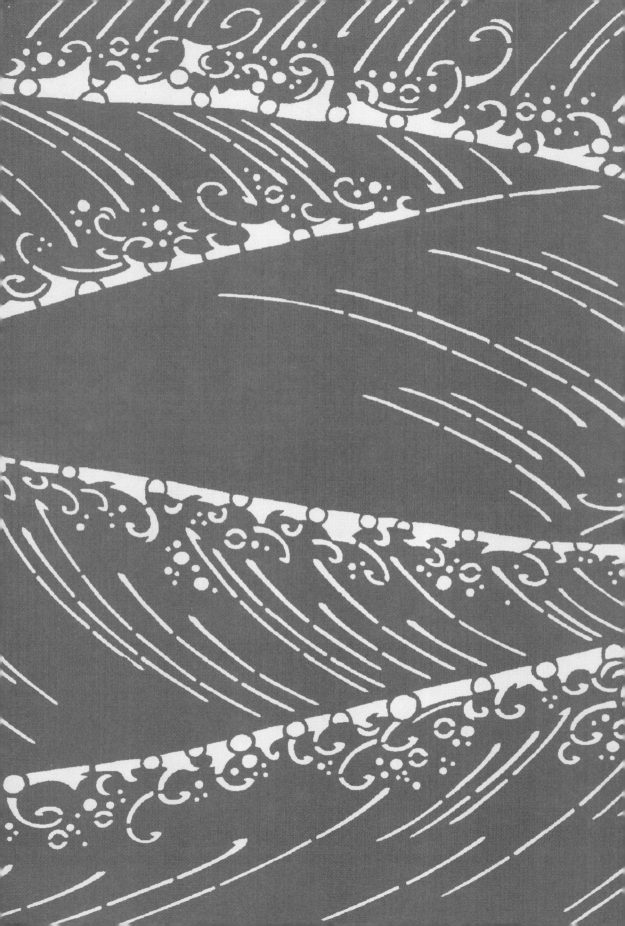

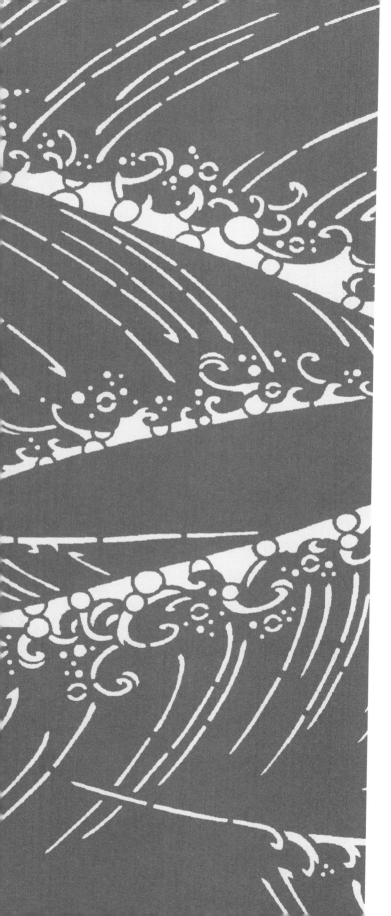

Mental Fitness

Complete Workouts
for Mind, Body,
and Soul

Michiko J. Rolek

with a foreword by
Leonard Cohen

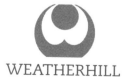

WEATHERHILL

First edition, 1996

Published by Weatherhill, Inc.
568 Broadway, Suite 705
New York, NY 10012

Library of Congress Cataloging-in-Publication Data

Rolek, Michiko J.
    Mental fitness: complete workouts for mind, body, and soul / Michiko J. Rolek
        p.   cm.
    Includes bibliographical references.
    ISBN 0-8348-0373-9 (pbk.)
    1. Mind and body. 2. Centering (Psychology) 3. Breathing exercises—therapeutic
    use. 4. Relaxation. I. Title.
    BF161.R75 1996
    158'.1—dc20   96-28110
                                                               CIP

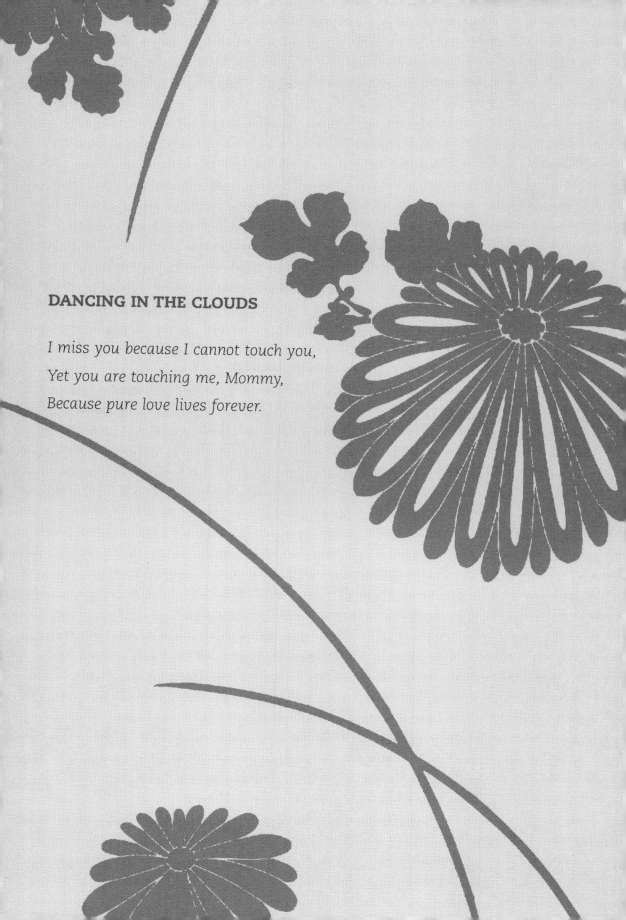

DANCING IN THE CLOUDS

I miss you because I cannot touch you,
Yet you are touching me, Mommy,
Because pure love lives forever.

CONTENTS

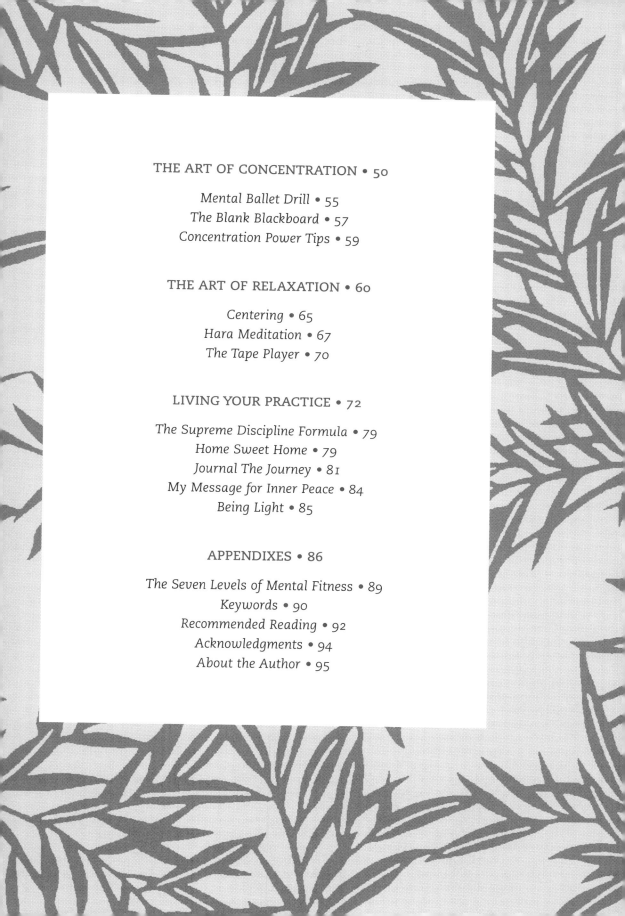

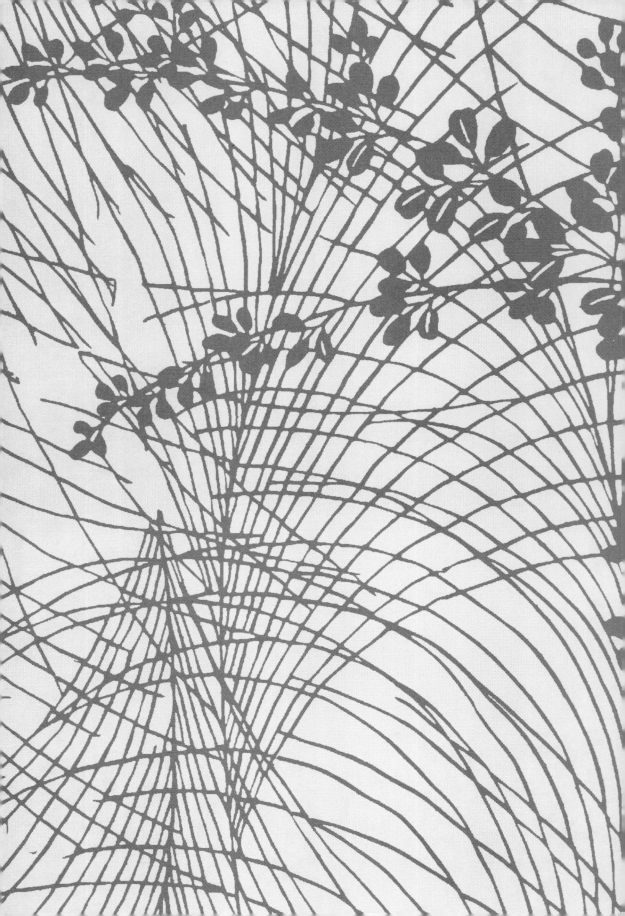

FOREWORD

My old teacher, Joshu Sasaki Roshi, has asked me to say a few words about the book which you are holding. He never really learned English, and he has forgotten much of his Japanese, but he knows a good thing when he sees it, and he wanted me to thank Michiko Rolek, on his behalf, for her very helpful instructions.

I live with a number of bewildered souls on a mountain in southern California. The place is called a Zen Center, and it probably is, but it is also a kind of hospital for people who have forgotten how to breathe, or sit, or stand, or walk. Michiko has developed a simple and effective approach to these fundamental activities. Some of us are breathing better already.

This workbook may not resolve the Burning Issues of Your Life, but you sure as hell can save yourself a lot of trouble by looking into it. You might even be able to skip having to visit a place like this, or if you are already in one, perhaps with this valuable information you can slip away.

In any case, we want to join Roshi in expressing our gratitude to Michiko for her kindness in presenting to us her manual on Mental Fitness. She has made some important matters wonderfully clear, and every page is informed by a sweet concern for the well-being of her reader.

Thank you.

> Jikan Eliezer
> a Mt. Baldy monk
> (Leonard Cohen)

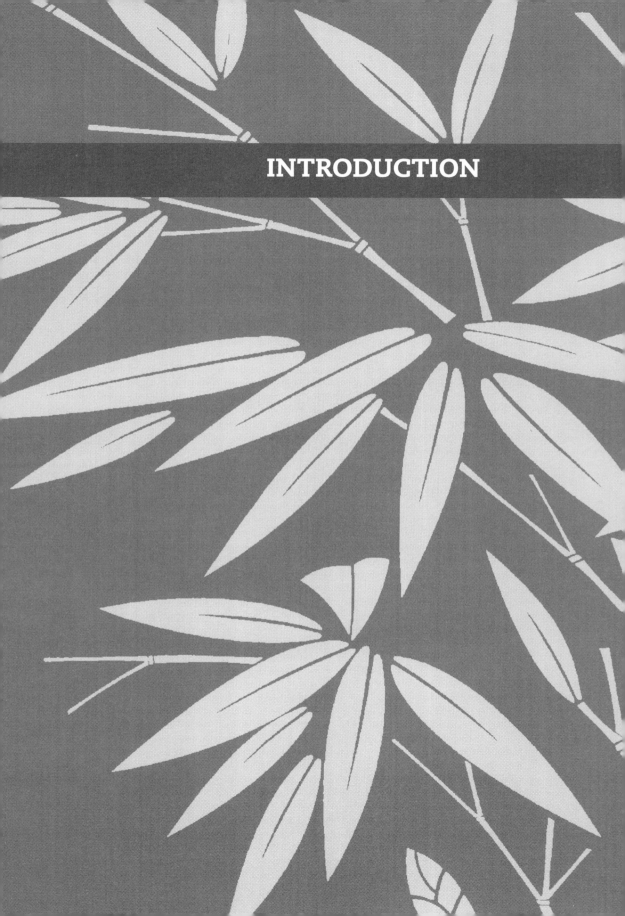

INTRODUCTION

We live in an information age. Most of us have read books on how to transform our lives and take charge of our future. We gain knowledge in this way, but knowledge is power only when we use it. Instead, we tend to get stuck in our thoughts, in the "non-doing" stage. True wisdom lies in applying what we know, so that knowledge and action become one. As Leo Buscaglia says, "To know, and not to do, is really not to know."

We learn by doing. This book is a formula, in the form of a training manual, for how to make this connection, to achieve unity of knowing and doing. We will address the brilliant basics, dealing only with the elements fundamental to your success. I want to inform you, not bore you with the superfluous. The material is user-friendly, easy for the beginner yet challenging enough for the more skilled student. You will learn effective techniques, ancient and modern, that are both fun and functional, and geared toward practice, not theory. When you practice them, you are building a foundation that will support you in any endeavor you choose. A commitment to this work will give you a great sense of accomplishment. Anything worthwhile takes dedication and self-discipline, eating bitter for the sweetness to come.

The Zen expression, "When the student is ready, the teacher will appear," communicates the attitude of willingness and openness that is necessary for Mental Fitness training. Since you have chosen this book to guide you on this path of discovery, I trust you are a student ready to grow from the inside out. I am honored to welcome you on this journey.

Wisdom has no cleverness in it.
It is pure and simple,
and when it is practiced
the results are obvious.

The Tao of Motherhood

There is magic in knowing that
transcends logic.

Wayne Dyer

WHAT IS MENTAL FITNESS?

You hold in your hands a tool kit that can change your life.

Mental Fitness is a system for strengthening yourself from the inside out. As I like to say, "Where the mind goes, the body follows." The essence of Mental Fitness is cultivating the soft, internally focused aspects of training, such as breathing, concentration, and centering, and incorporating them into your daily life. Through exercises such as the Centered Breath, the Centered Stance, and Hara Meditation, you will learn how to develop these fundamental skills.

Mental Fitness is an inner workout: an absolute necessity if you are to function at your best. It will rejuvenate your entire system and develop pure inner energy that will bring you greater results on all levels, enabling you to focus on and follow through with your heart's desire.

Mental Fitness gives you a training edge. Through it, you will cultivate the qualities of concentration, awareness, and discipline; qualities that establish a readiness for action and achievement. Through it you will realize fitness of mind, body, and soul. This is real power, power that lasts.

Mental Fitness is about resilience: keeping your head strong and your vision clear. Staying focused on your vision will carry you through difficult times. When setbacks occur, it will be easier to bounce back on track and overcome obstacles. Just visualize it, believe it, and you will achieve it—by focusing on the process, not the product.

Best of all, getting Mentally Fit can be a private experience. You can do it anywhere, at any time, and no one else will be aware that you are fine-tuning your mind and body for greater energy and awareness.

*Nothing is more powerful
and creative than emptiness.*

Lao Tzu

*The great man is he who
does not lose the child's heart.*

Mencius

*I hear and I forget.
I see and I remember.
I do and I understand.*

Chinese Proverb

EMPTY YOUR CUP

To establish the Beginners' Mindset for optimum learning and transformation, we must first empty our ego minds—that part of us also known as the chattering mind, that doubts and offers resistance. We must let go of past notions and limitations that are depleting us rather than nourishing us.

In Zen, this is called the Don't-Know mind. It is like becoming a child again. If we already know, or think we know something, how can we learn anything new? Our cup is full. Unless we come to the learning process with emptiness, how can we receive anything?

By opening and stretching your mind, you become more receptive, inviting in new ideas and attitudes to build your Mental Fitness and transform your life.

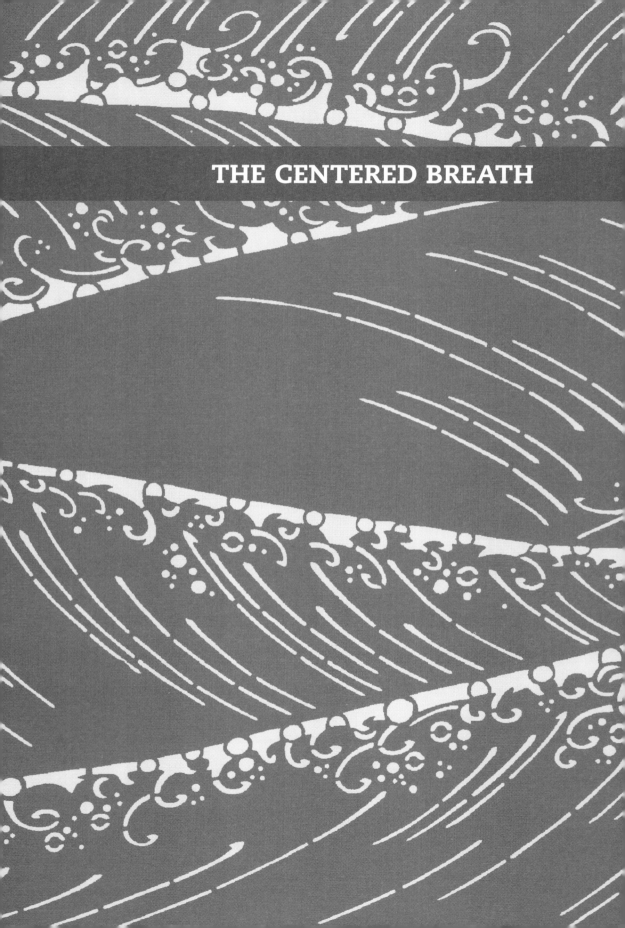

THE CENTERED BREATH

STACKING BOOKS

An Imagery Exercise

This illustration will help you to visualize the mechanics of the Deluxe Breath Technique.

Imagine stacking a pile of books. Place one book on top of another until you have built a tall stack. The first book you placed is at the bottom of the stack and the last book is on the top.

Now, unstack the books, one at a time. You must start at the top of the pile and work your way to the bottom.

As you do the Deluxe Breath Technique, think of your breath as this pile of books that you must steadily stack and unstack.

Inhalation is like the process of stacking. Start the air at the bottom, deep into the cradle of your hara. Slowly "stack" your breath all the way up to your collarbones.

Exhalation is the process of unstacking. Starting from the top, slowly "unstack" your breath from the collarbones to the lower abdomen.

THE LONG BREATH OUT

Out with the old, in with the new. That's what breathing is all about.

We all know the importance of breathing in. If we don't do it, we die. Our bodies need oxygen to survive.

Breathing out is equally important. When you breathe out fully, the next inhalation is effortless. It is during the exhalation phase that we eliminate impurities, toxins, and garbage energy from our system. Without this purifying process, our bodies would shut down.

The Long Breath Out, also known as Zen Breathing, is simply extending the duration of time that you exhale. The longer we exhale, the more we benefit.

Aside from its cleansing benefits, The Long Breath Out also

- Strengthens the lower abdomen.

- Decreases upper body tension.

- Clears the mind and helps you relax.

- Focuses and directs your energy.

- Releases power to activate muscles.

Holding your breath locks tension into your body and causes the mind to spin with anxiety. So remember, in any tight situation, "When in doubt, Long Breath Out."

BREATHING OPTIONS

When doing these exercises, intended to increase lung capacity, work at your fitness level. Always modify. Listen to your body, and never force or strain. The key is feeling comfortable. Counting helps you concentrate and keep your mind focused on your breathing.

The Centered Breath with Counting

1. Inhale slowly, 4 counts.

2. Pause, holding the breath comfortably, up to 4 counts.

3. Exhale evenly and smoothly, 4 counts.

Get comfortable breathing in and out rhythmically. Then try it with the Long Breath Out at a 2:1 ratio. For example, breathe in for 3 to 5 counts, then breathe out for 6 to 10 counts.

The Deluxe Breath with Counting

1. Breathe into the lower abdomen on a count of 1... 2... Allow the breath to rise up inside your rib cage and up to the collarbones on counts 3... 4... 5...

2. Pause, hold the breath comfortably, up to 5 counts.

3. Slowly breathe out from top to bottom. Start from the collarbones on counts 1... 2... 3... Keep it moving smoothly and steadily downward, 4... 5... 6... Pull in the lower abdomen on counts 7... 8... 9... 10...

Build up slowly to a full, deep inhalation and a long, extended exhalation. Those of you with more experience can inhale more deeply and exhale longer.

As we energize our bellies,
we strengthen our physical connection
to our spiritual source.

Lisa Sarasohn

The breath is the ultimate key
to controlling fear and anxiety.

Andy Caponigro

THE SEA WIND BREATH TECHNIQUE

I like to think of diaphragmatic breathing as classical respiration.

After all, most classically trained singers and wind instrumentalists breathe from their hara or gut for the tremendous energy and optimal performance it gives them.

To experience this harmony, listen inwardly to the ebb and flow of your breath with the Sea Wind Technique. The breath is sweet, internal music.

The basis of this technique comes from the yogic breathing method known as Ujjayi, which means "to produce a sound." It increases body heat, awakening the muscles and boosting the metabolism. The Sea Wind Technique also facilitates concentration and endurance.

1. Take a few Centered Breaths to relax all over.

2. Whisper, deep in your throat, the hollow sound "HA," keeping your mouth open while exhaling. On inhalation make the sound "SA." Note the air touching the back of your throat. This should feel like a breath of soft, cool, sea wind. Repeat this step until you are comfortable with it.

3. Continue to make the sounds on inhalation and exhalation, only now with your mouth closed. Rest your tongue on the roof of your mouth or behind the bottom front teeth.

4. Listen to the soothing, sea wind sound of your breath and stay in this forward-flowing rhythm. Remain inwardly calm and take your time.

Practice for 5–15 minutes.

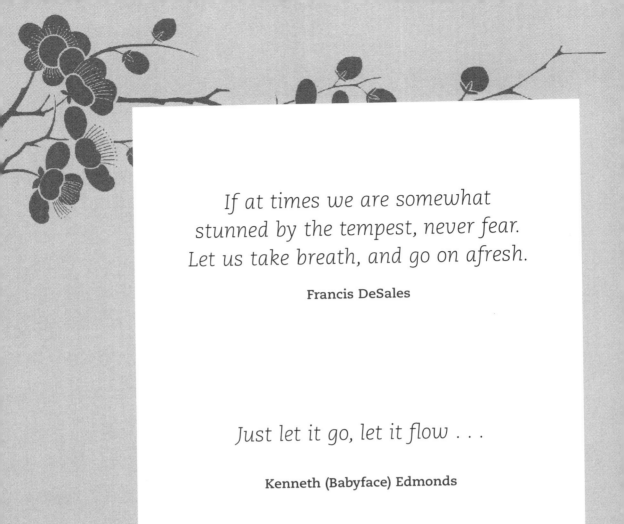

*If at times we are somewhat
stunned by the tempest, never fear.
Let us take breath, and go on afresh.*

Francis DeSales

Just let it go, let it flow . . .

Kenneth (Babyface) Edmonds

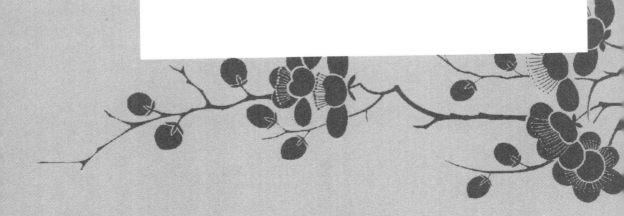

GOING WITH THE FLOW BREATH TECHNIQUE

This technique will activate your right-brain qualities, such as intuition and creativity, while keeping the anxiety cycle in check. It will promote feelings of compassion and awaken your free spirit.

1. Begin with a few easy Sea Wind breaths through both nostrils.

2. Close your right nostril with your index finger and exhale slowly and completely through your left nostril. (Do not use the Sea Wind Breath on your exhalation.)

3. Breathe in through both nostrils, listening to the Sea Wind sound.

4. Close off your left nostril with your index finger and exhale slowly and completely through your right nostril.

5. Continue alternating nostrils with each Long Breath Out. Sense each exhalation like a long, flowing silk ribbon.

   Practice for 5–10 minutes.

For a Quick Mental Tune-up to sharpen concentration, check out this baby-simple version of alternate nostril breathing:

1. Close your right nostril with your right index finger. Breathe out and in deeply through the left nostril three times. Do it slowly.

2. Now close the left nostril with your right or left hand and breathe out and in through the right nostril three times.

3. Place both hands in your lap, palms up, and breathe out and in deeply through both nostrils. Notice feeling energized, cool, and confident in nine easy breaths.

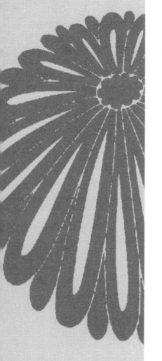

*Behold, I will cause
breath to enter into you,
and ye shall live.*

Ezekiel 37:5

*And the Lord God formed man
of the dust of the ground,
and breathed into his nostrils
the breath of life;
and man became a living soul.*

Genesis 2:7

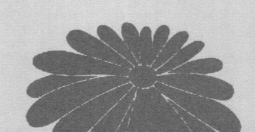

BREATH POWER TIPS

Any time. Any place. The magic of breath work is that you can do it anywhere, regardless of what you are doing. Rush-hour traffic, long lines at the grocery store. Take advantage of these precious moments. Breathe.

Start at your level. The key is to feel comfortable. Never force or strain. Breathe as deeply as you can. Exhale as long as you can. The main thing is to do what you can.

The Energy Boost. Need a lift? Take a few deep Centered Breaths. Concentrate on the inhalation. Oxygen wakes up those tired cells. Remember, inhalation generates breath energy. It is active or Yang.

Chill Out. Feeling stressed? Burned out? Here's a quick stress buster. Close your eyes and take three Centered Breaths. Concentrate on the Long Breath Out. Exhalation frees your mind, promotes relaxation and focuses your energy. It is passive or Yin.

Enjoy the Great Outdoors. Take a trip to the mountains or a walk on the beach. Not only is the fresh air rejuvenating, but a little exercise and change of scenery will do wonders for you.

Stop, Look & Listen. Be mindful. Become aware of your breathing patterns throughout the day. The goal is to breathe more deeply, more consistently.

Practice Makes Perfect. As with developing any skill, proper breathing techniques take patience and persistence. With focused practice, Centered Breathing will become second nature to you within a month.

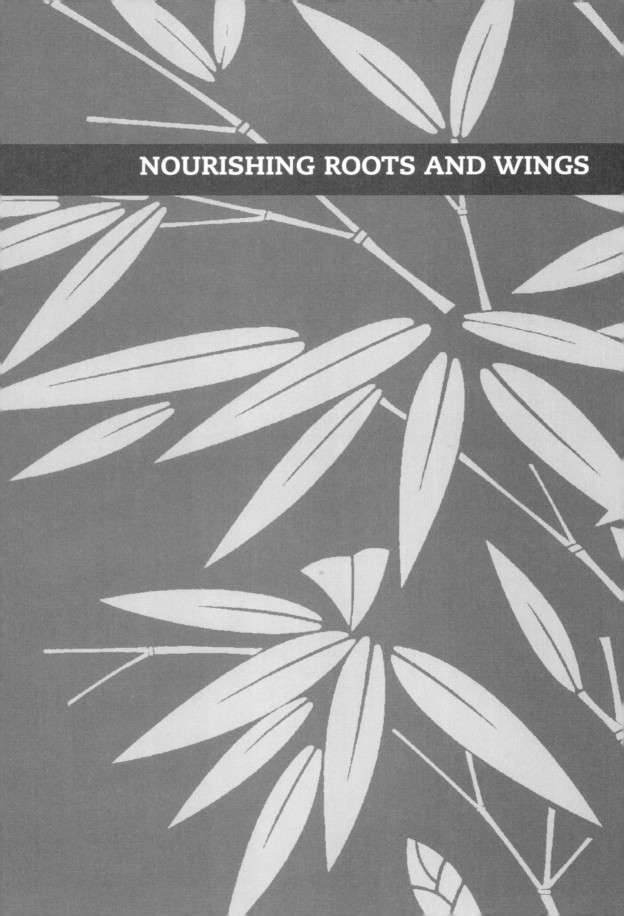

NOURISHING ROOTS AND WINGS

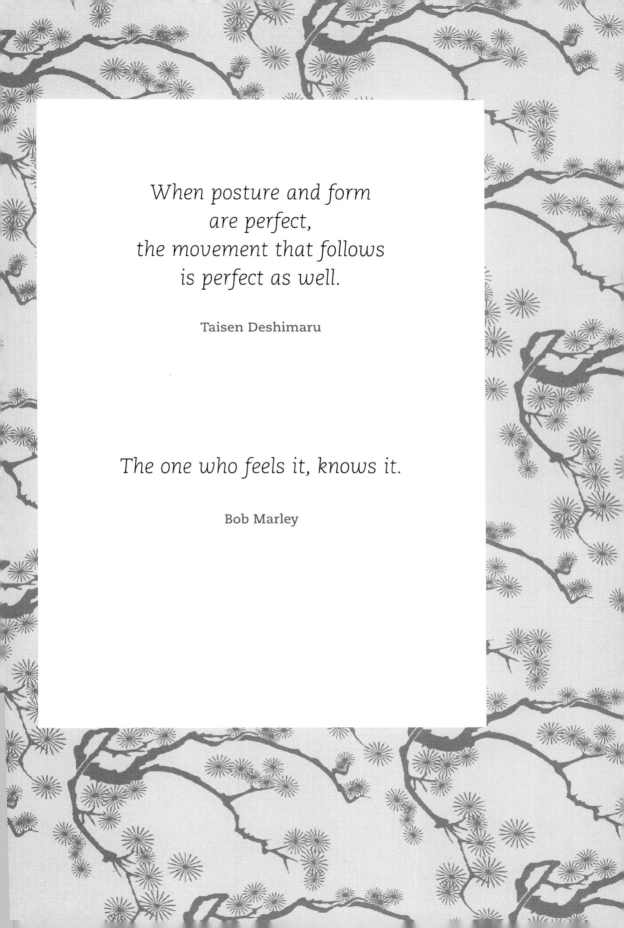

When posture and form
are perfect,
the movement that follows
is perfect as well.

Taisen Deshimaru

The one who feels it, knows it.

Bob Marley

THE CENTERED STANCE

These are the building blocks of good posture.

Take them one at a time. Become comfortable with each one before moving to the next. When you are aware of each sensation, slowly link them together to achieve the Centered Stance.

- Stand with your feet a shoulder width apart. Lengthen and spread your toes. Relax into the floor, sinking deep roots, inch by inch. Feel as if the bottoms of your feet are magnetized to the earth. Keep your weight even on both feet.

- Straighten your legs by lifting your thigh muscles upward, or softly bend your knees, keeping them pointed in the direction of the middle toes.

- Center your pelvis. Tuck it in slightly by lifting the pubic bone. This straightens the lower spine. Do not over-tuck. The bottom of your hips should be directly over the centers of your feet.

- Your hara should become firm as an iron ball, keeping your center of gravity low. Breathe deeply and continuously. As you exhale, press your navel inward and upward towards your spine.

- Lift and expand your rib cage from within. Sense it like a bell hanging inside you. Don't stick out your chest; keep it relaxed.

- The shoulders should be relaxed and forward, parallel to your hips. Feel them spreading, soft and wide, like wings.

- Soften and tuck in your chin to elevate the crown of your head. This aligns your head with your spine and stretches the back of your neck. Your chin should be parallel to the floor. Feel as if you are suspended from above.

Touchstone for Martial Artists and Dancers. The lower spine must be straight and deeply rooted in order to achieve the proper upper thigh rotation known as turn-out. This torque action is empowered by centering the pelvis, which in turn lowers the center of gravity. This is the touchstone for improved balance. Turning out from the hip joints also prevents knee and ankle injuries.

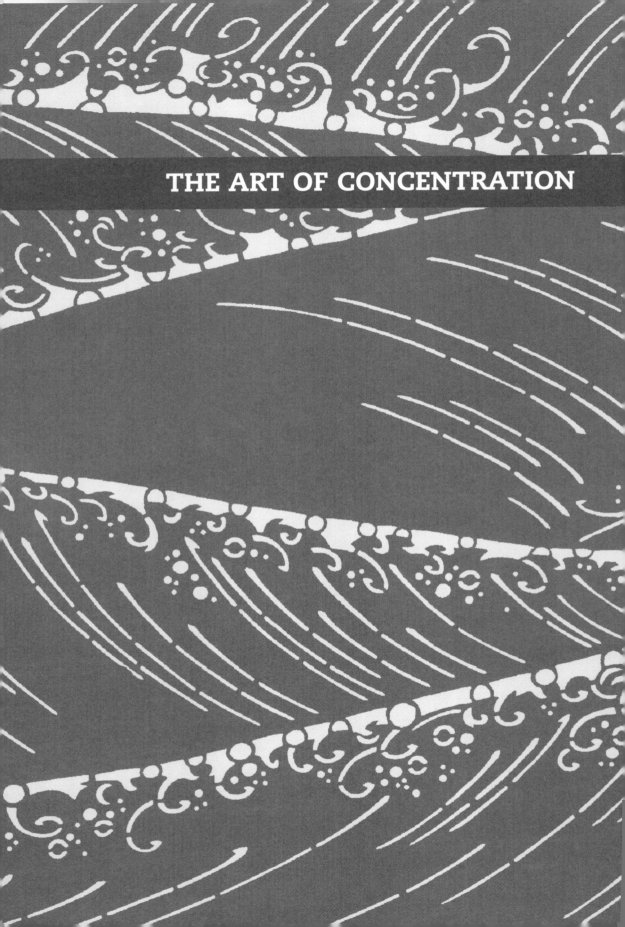

THE ART OF CONCENTRATION

MENTAL BALLET DRILL

The following three-part drill is intended to strengthen your concentration. Each part develops a different skill.

Practice them one at a time.

Before beginning each step, sit comfortably upright. Close your eyes. Rest your hands on your lap. Take a few Centered Breaths and settle into a steady rhythm. Centered Breathing sets the stage for ideal concentration.

Focus

- Place your attention on your Third Eye, known in yoga as the Ajna Chakra or Soul Center. It is located deep inside your forehead at a still point between your two eyebrows. This centered-up feeling brings a calm yet alert state of being.

- Count down from 5 to 1. Each time you exhale, mentally see and feel the number, one at a time. Stay focused on the number and say it to yourself silently while centering down with each Long Breath Out. Repeat as often as you like. Counting disciplines the mind to stay focused, which strengthens the concentration.

Fluidity

- Once you have settled into a focused mindset, it is time to build up your attention span. This is accomplished through continuous awareness of the breath and counting.

- Mentally count down from 25 to 1, sensing each number in your mind's eye. Keep your attention focused on the numbers and just breathe naturally. Let it flow.

- If your mind drifts, bring your attention back to your breath and begin counting again from 25 to 1.

You will be "in the flow" when you can count from 25 to 1 without distraction.

Agility

Mental agility is activated when your mind wanders and you instantly bring it back into the present moment.

- With your eyes closed, center up and count down from 5 to 1. As you exhale, sense the numbers one at a time, as you did in the focus exercise.

- Now, open your eyes and zero in on an object, gazing at it momentarily.

- Close your eyes again and return to counting down from 5 to 1.

- To develop catlike readiness, practice shifting your attention back and forth in this way.

The essence of mental agility is being able to downshift into the moment quickly and easily. Breath awareness always gives us a choice to transform negative reactions and responses into simple, quiet observation, which is positive.

THE BLANK BLACKBOARD

An Imagery Exercise

Do you remember the big blackboards they had at the front of the classroom when you were in school? The teacher would write ideas and notes all over it. When it was full, she would take an eraser and clear the board.

Imagine using a mental eraser in the same way in order to clear your mind to concentrate.

Close your eyes and center up between your eyebrows. In your mind's eye, imagine a blank blackboard.

Sitting comfortably upright, take a few deep Centered Breaths. Focus on your breathing.

Whenever a thought or distraction pops into your mind, see yourself erasing your blackboard. Use big, sweeping strokes with each Long Breath Out.

Each time your mental blackboard is erased, the thoughts are released. Become familiar with the clear space you have created. Rest in it for as long as you feel comfortable. Experience this quietly alert state.

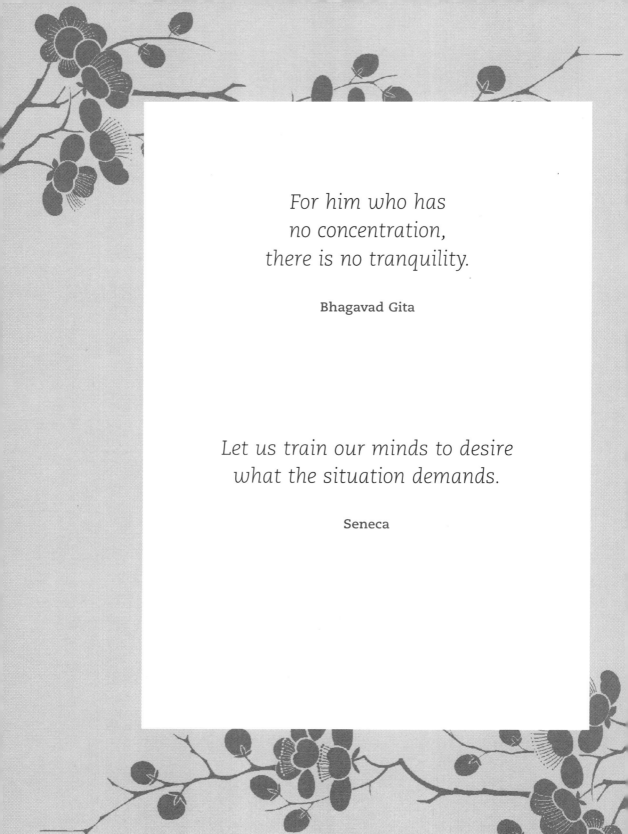

*For him who has
no concentration,
there is no tranquility.*

Bhagavad Gita

*Let us train our minds to desire
what the situation demands.*

Seneca

CONCENTRATION POWER TIPS

Details, Details, Details. Take a moment, wherever you are, and look at something: a painting, a building, a tree. Really look at it. Become aware of as many details as you can see: the colors, the textures, the obvious, the hidden. This attentiveness sharpens your focus so that you don't just look, but really see.

Quality, Not Quantity. A little concentration goes a long way. Fifteen minutes of a focused activity is more effective than two hours of scattered energy and boredom. Concentration enables you to spend your time, not waste it.

Pleasure Principle. When you like an activity, you can be totally absorbed in it for hours. Capture the essence by doing more of what you enjoy. Focusing on what you like builds your concentration, so that tasks you enjoy less can still get done.

Mindfulness. You can only think one thought at a time, so why not be here, now. Developing concentration skills enables you to focus your mind in the moment. Release what has happened in the past or what might happen in the future. Your place of power is always in the present.

Enjoy the Journey. Developing concentration takes practice. Commit and follow through all the way. Regarding our work as play helps us to focus and flow better.

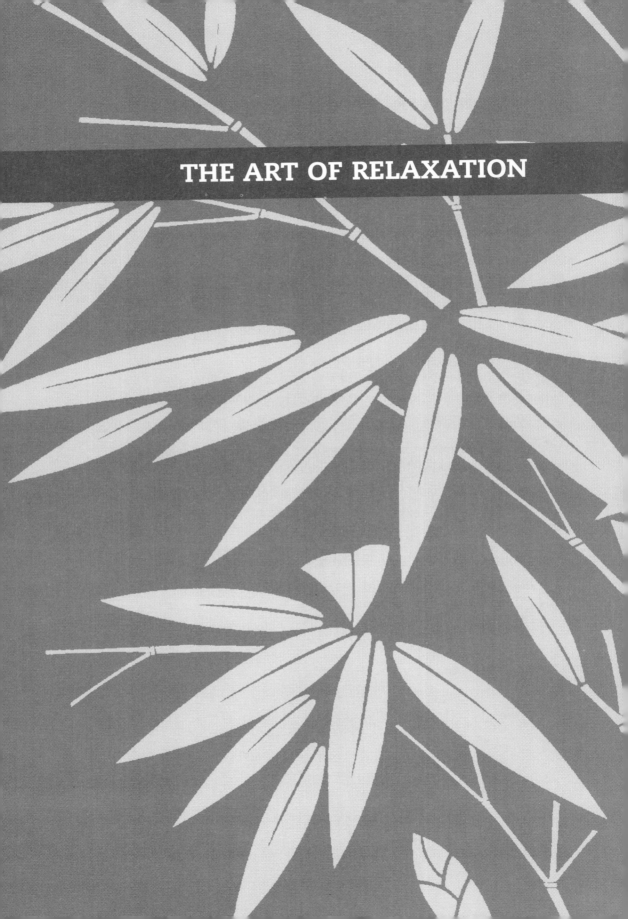

THE ART OF RELAXATION

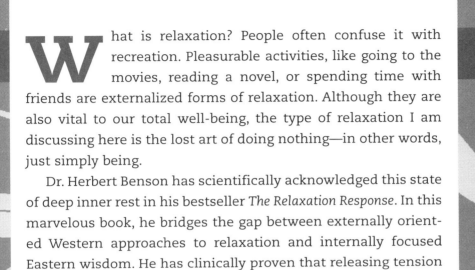

What is relaxation? People often confuse it with recreation. Pleasurable activities, like going to the movies, reading a novel, or spending time with friends are externalized forms of relaxation. Although they are also vital to our total well-being, the type of relaxation I am discussing here is the lost art of doing nothing—in other words, just simply being.

Dr. Herbert Benson has scientifically acknowledged this state of deep inner rest in his bestseller *The Relaxation Response*. In this marvelous book, he bridges the gap between externally oriented Western approaches to relaxation and internally focused Eastern wisdom. He has clinically proven that releasing tension triggers a calming response in our mind and body from which a sense of inner peace naturally follows.

The Latin root of "relax" simply means "to let go." When we let go of unnecessary stress and regulate our nervous system through Centered Breathing, we find our way into the meditative state of relaxation.

The dictionary defines stress as placing emphasis or pressure on something. Stress, in itself, is not the problem. The problem is how we interpret and respond to it. Some people thrive on pressure and deadlines, and are invigorated by the challenge; others simply feel threatened and overwhelmed.

People who can handle pressure know how to manage their emotional states efficiently and effectively. This requires courage, an invisible sense of trust, and a positive, focused attitude. I call this "grace under pressure." It is only when we relax, by using the Long Breath Out, that we can access this reservoir of personal power in any challenging situation.

On the other hand, the worry-hurry stress response of fight or flight builds anxiety that can escalate into exhausting, agonizing tension. These symptoms can be alleviated through proper relaxation technique. When we notice that our minds are spinning anxiously and our bodies are tight, we can breathe out the toxic tension and feel the relief of letting go.

Scientific research shows that if we are relaxed, negative feelings such as anger, fear, and insecurity are not given the energy or power to upset us. Relaxation loosens the emotional ropes that once tied us up. We must acknowledge that what we resist persists to bother us— and that we can choose to let go of the ego's resistance.

The word release is derived from the same source as relax, and implies setting something free. Relaxing is the letting go of muscular tension, and releasing is the letting go of thoughts, emotions, and anything else that needs to be mentally set free. It is this combination of mental release with physical relaxation and centering that allows us to experience true inner peace.

Moving towards the center is a meditative process. Through meditation we learn to sit still and quiet the mind by relaxing and listening. Centering is the ability to direct the mental focus from the outer world to our inner world. Once again, it is the Centered Breath that makes true relaxation possible. Breathing deeply to the core and concentrating on the Long Breath Out slows the spinning mind, releases tension throughout the body, and triggers our natural relaxation response. The choice is ours to make. Remain centered, and you can act from calmness rather than reacting with anxiety.

When we relax, it is like the kinks being loosened out of a hose. Our energy can now flow freely, without obstruction. Naura Hayden says that tension is nothing more than trapped energy, or talent that is stuck. Cyberphysiology pioneer José Silva concluded that since the brain is an electrical system, the optimal circuit is the one with the least resistance or static. The brain is actually more energetic when it is less active or noisy.

This lowered brain-wave activity is called the alpha frequency and is known to promote calm, lucid concentration. When we totally relax from head to toe, entering this alpha state, the mind receives and stores more information. In alpha, the right, intuitive hemisphere of the brain is turned on. Some of the qualities of your right brain are spiritual insight, music, healing ability, and creative imagination. Dynamic energy is also accessed from your subconscious right brain. By saying "yes" to letting go of tension, you give yourself permission to totally relax, sink deeper into yourself, and awaken the creative free spirit inside of you.

With the relaxation skills you are about to learn, you can clear away any obstruction that stands in your way, so that you are able to flow forward and take action. Take note that it is not hard work that drains our energy, but emotional turbulence. According to Norman Vincent Peale's classic book *The Power of Positive Thinking*, inventor Thomas Edison had constant energy and only needed three to five hours of sleep a night. When asked why this was so, he said he drew his tremendous energy from emotional self-mastery and the ability to relax completely. The key to relaxation is simple: we must monitor doubt and constantly refocus to stay positive.

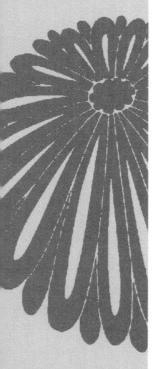

To study the Buddha Way
is to study the self.
To study the self is to forget the self.
To forget the self is to be enlightened
by the ten thousand things.

Dogen Zenji

Quiet minds cannot
be perplexed or frightened,
but go on in fortune or misfortune
at their own private pace,
like a clock during a thunderstorm.

Robert Louis Stevenson

Know thyself, and thou shalt
know the universe.

Socrates

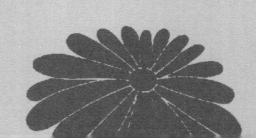

CENTERING

Every day, we are faced with unexpected challenges and tensions. We are constantly pulled away from our sense of center and, at times, thrown off balance.

True relaxation comes by focusing our minds inward and returning to our vital center, or hara. This restores balance and harmony to our nervous system. Centering establishes an inner calm that is comfortable and steady, regardless of outer circumstances. With an awareness of center, we build our inner strength. A quiet mind is a confident mind.

The samurai of medieval Japan knew the importance and power of this simple fact. They would spend countless hours strengthening their hara through breath control and the sitting meditation known as Zazen. Borrowing from my samurai roots, I would now like to share with you a modified version of this sitting meditation. It will embody most of the techniques I have shared with you in this handbook.

This meditation exercise introduces, in a neutral manner, the art of centering. Centering allows your mind and body to become unified. Like the great samurai, you will be strengthening your hara or guts: developing your ability to stay calm, energized, and fearless in any situation that life can throw your way. This centering discipline is the code to becoming a peaceful or spiritual warrior. By releasing the need for outer approval and control, the true warrior goes home within and discovers self-discipline and self-approval. Alan Watts embraced this idea when he asked us, "If you do not get it from yourself, where will you go for it?"

Nowhere can man find
a quieter or more
untroubled retreat
than in his own soul.

Marcus Aurelius

Meditation, then, is bringing
the mind home.

Sogyal Rinpoche

HARA MEDITATION

Find a place to get comfortable for 5 to 20 minutes, a place that is as quiet as possible and free from distractions. Sit deep and still in a chair, or cross-legged on the floor. Being still naturally dissolves restless sensations.

Straighten your spine by pressing your crown upward away from your shoulders. Imagine your head to be a sunflower on a long stem. To straighten your lower spine, root your rear end firmly and tip your pelvis forward, feeling your torso rise from the cradle of your hips. If necessary, sit on a cushion or rolled-up towel to help you maintain this position.

Give your body permission to relax all over. Place your hands on your lap, left palm resting upward in the right palm, with the thumbs lightly touching if you choose. Keep your lower abdomen firm by breathing deep and exhaling long. Assume an inner smile by gently turning up the corners of your mouth. Place your tongue on the roof of your mouth.

Allow your eyes to close and center up between your eyebrows, or leave them partially open, softly gazing forward at a point a few feet ahead of you. Mentally watch your Centered Breath coming and going. Inhale, the tummy rises. Exhale, the tummy falls.

Zero in on your Long Breath Out. This will flush and drain upper body tension. If you get drowsy, take a few deep inhalations to awaken and send an extra boost of oxygen to your brain.

Stay focused on your Centered Breath and your upright posture. Give yourself permission to sink deeper, like a wave becoming one with the depths of the ocean.

As you rest in your Centered Breath flow, allow it to become effortless. Let your body do it for you.

After a few moments, become aware of your internal bodily sensations: the drumbeat of your heart, the rhythm and the tingling flow of oxygenated blood bringing warmth to your hara and coolness to your forehead. Even though you are motionless, there is an inner dance of constant cellular motion.

Take a moment to experience your spine moving with the flow of your breath. It is like a sea horse riding the breath waves. When you inhale, your spine elongates and gently arches. When you exhale, your spine rounds like the letter C as your tummy pulls inward. Become aware of these very subtle, internal movements.

You are tuning into your body's natural wisdom and learning to trust it. Maintain an attitude of gratitude for the harmonious, internal activity of your body.

When your attention diverts or your mind wanders, gently return to your breath. Restless sensations, doubts, and distractions are normal. By keeping a let-it-happen attitude, they will dissolve easily, as your mind is being trained not to entertain them. Too much effort interferes and tenses you up. Instead, let your thoughts float by like dancing clouds. Be aware of their presence but not influenced by them. Observing your thoughts and not reacting to them teaches you tranquil detachment while you establish a clear mind and peaceful heart.

To end your meditation, sit quietly alert, do nothing, and be still. Notice feeling more self-connected and peaceful. You have returned to your spiritual source. Coming home to your true nature puts you back in touch with your unity with divinity. As the scripture says, "Be still and know that I am God within you." (Psalms 46:10)

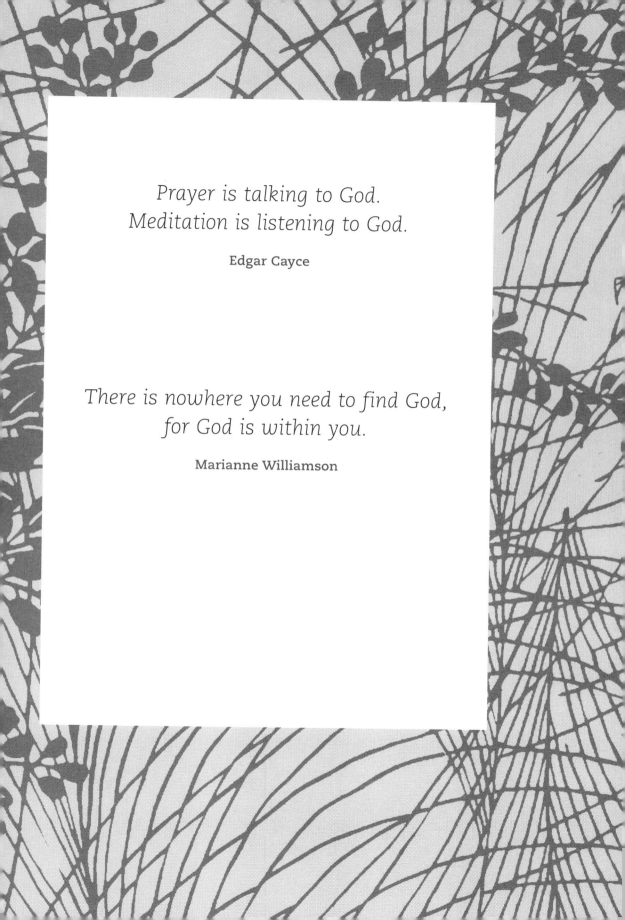

Prayer is talking to God.
Meditation is listening to God.

Edgar Cayce

There is nowhere you need to find God,
for God is within you.

Marianne Williamson

THE TAPE PLAYER

An Imagery Exercise

Take a look at the buttons on a tape player.

There is the REWIND *button, so we can play something over and over again. There is the* FAST FORWARD *button, so we can jump ahead. There is the* PAUSE *button, which brings everything to a standstill. Not quite stopped and not quite playing, frozen in time.*

Sometimes our minds tend to spin like the drive wheels on our players.

We REWIND, *spinning into the past, reliving something that already has happened. We* FAST FORWARD, *spinning into the future, worrying about things that might be. Sometimes, we are on* PAUSE. *Just plain stuck.*

Meditation helps us to become more mindful, centered in the present moment. We want to keep our mind's tape player always in the PLAY *mode. For only the* PLAY *button allows us to experience everything as it is happening now.*

In your mind's eye, visualize your mental tape player. Anytime you are distracted or your mind strays, use your Long Breath Out to bring you back to center. To stretch your imagination further, pretend you are wearing headphones and listen inwardly to your breath flow.

Press the PLAY *button and be here now!*

*The present moment
is a powerful Goddess.*

Goethe

*Live each present moment
completely and the future
will take care of itself.*

Paramahansa Yogananda

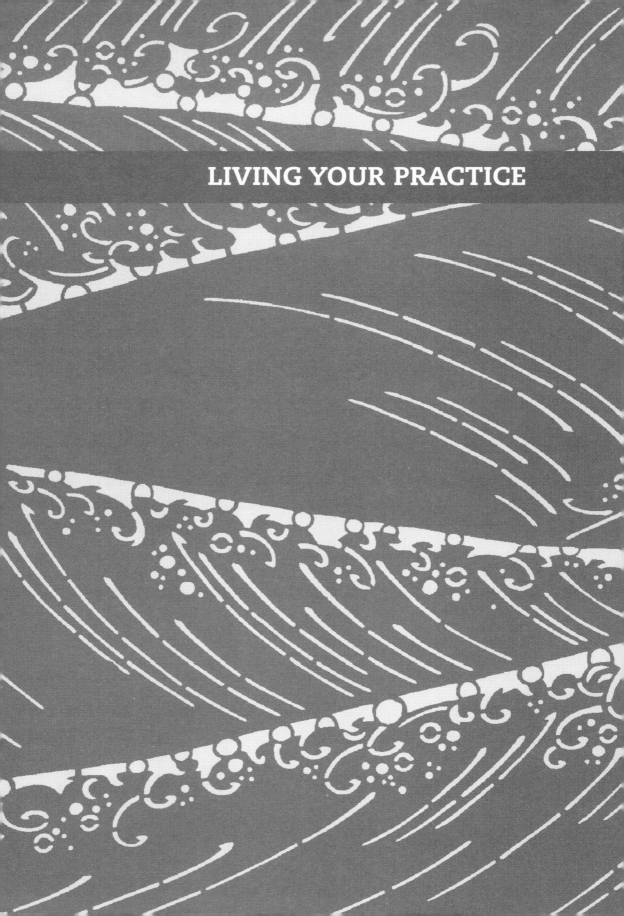

LIVING YOUR PRACTICE

You have now finished reading about a few basic techniques that will help improve the quality of your life. First things first. Learn it, now use it. Getting good at anything requires developing good mental habits and discipline through patience, practice, and persistence. Mental Fitness is no different. It is simple, but not easy.

However, there is one major advantage. Mental Fitness allows you to take your show on the road. Wherever you go, whatever you do, the principles go with you. Mental Fitness can and should be practiced at any time and in any place. When I heard how much basketball superstar Michael Jordan loves to practice, the reality of his greatness became clearer to me. Phil Jackson, head coach of the Chicago Bulls, calls Jordan's playing style "The Zen of Air." He proves that focusing on form and practice unleashes our magic and transforms us.

Nobody can practice all the time, or would want to, for that matter. We all have busy lives with many things to do, and there never seems to be enough time in the day. But you must make the time. You are worth it. I've discovered that when we take our time, we have enough of it. It is when we rush that we are always out of it. Bruce Lee called this "slowing down to go faster," which is like a Zen koan or riddle.

It would be ideal if you could set aside a half-hour to an hour at the beginning and the end of each day to devote solely to your practice. Setting aside this quiet time for yourself is very important to your total health and well-being. But for many people, even this may be asking too much.

There is a way, however, that allows you to master the techniques of Mental Fitness without interrupting your busy schedule. I call this Living Your Practice. The key is awareness: being tuned in. Awareness of the principles set out in this book. Awareness of your breath and posture. Awareness of your thoughts and feelings. In essence, embracing each present moment with all-out attention. In his book *Sacred Hoops*, Phil Jackson shares this outlook of "awareness is everything." His approach—bringing Eastern concepts into a Western sport to create what he calls Mindful Basketball—is related to our efforts at playing to win in the game of life. But I see winning as reaching toward a goal, not simply getting there; an attitude that keeps us centered and less stressful.

Whenever we notice ourselves doing something that is not beneficial to our Mental Fitness, we can change it. If you catch yourself slouched over your desk, sit upright. If you see your mind spinning anxiously, wondering "what if...," focus on your breath and return to your center. Only through self-awareness do we have the power to alter our mental state. We cannot stop the waves of change, but we can ride them on our mental surfboards.

Now that you are informed about the nuts and bolts of how to generate unity of mind, body, and soul, let's connect the dots and finish the picture of how we can practice the principles we have learned in this handbook and incorporate them into our everyday lives. It has been said that order is the first rule of Heaven. Keeping this in mind, let's start at the beginning.

The Centered Breath is your vital path to active self-mastery. It is the golden silk thread running through all the exercises in this book. Paying attention to the breath and nurturing it is the essence of your practice, and should be your first priority. Practice your breathing every opportunity you get; it is that important. Whenever the thought of breathing comes to mind, take a few deep Centered Breaths. No matter where you are or what you are doing, there is always time for a quick breath check. While taking a shower, driving to work, or even talking on the telephone, it only takes a few seconds. Make sure you are breathing abdominally. If not, make the adjustment.

Remember, the more you are aware of your mind and body, the more you can benefit from the power of your breath. If you find yourself getting anxious and tense, you can dissolve these feelings with the Going With the Flow Technique. If you could use some get-up-and-go, try the Deluxe Breath. To sharpen your concentration, the Quick Mental Tune-up in nine breaths is an option. As author Stuart Wilde reminds us, self-discipline quiets the mind and raises our energy levels.

You are the pilot of your breath, and it is always there for you. Use it and experience its healing effects, such as a slower heart rate and lower blood pressure. Breathing right also increases the production of the pleasure hormones known as endorphins. Feeling wonderful comes naturally when you develop the healthful habit of diaphragmatic breathing.

Nourishing Roots and Wings is an ongoing process. Like watering a plant, your posture needs constant attention. With awareness, you will find many opportunities to practice throughout the day. Long lines at the bank or grocery store are great places to work on standing posture. Besides, if you are focusing on your alignment, the lines won't seem as long. Eating dinner, working at your desk, or even watching videos from your favorite chair—whenever you sit down—think of hanging from your hook in the sky. Not only will you improve your posture, you will feel more comfortable.

The more you take notice of your posture and correct it, the stronger your alignment becomes. Soon, with your center firm, it becomes effortless, and you will feel the dignity and grace that can be yours for a lifetime.

The Art of Concentration should also become part of your daily routine. The key to living your practice is simply this: whatever you do, experiment with doing it more mindfully. Pay complete attention to your moment-to-moment experiences.

Mindfulness can be a celebration of the senses. When you sit down to eat, shut off the television and put down the newspaper. Don't just devour your food, experience the meal. Take note of the food in front of you; the colors, the smells, the temperature. Eat slowly and really taste every bite. This simple activity will not only help you develop your mindfulness, it will also naturally aid your digestive process.

Listening is another great way to live the practice of concentration. Pay attention to the sounds around you. If you are having a conversation, really hear what the other person is saying. If the radio is on, listen to every word of your favorite song.

Your objective should be to do one thing or think one thought at a time, even if you have lots of things to do. Success coach Rita Davenport says, "If you want to catch a rabbit, don't chase after nine at the same time." We cannot travel in two directions simultaneously, nor can our minds think two thoughts at once. When you recognize this, you can downshift back to center, redirect your focus, and do what must be done. Training the mind is like training a muscle: it needs to be exercised consistently to keep it strong and flexible.

The foundation of emotional self-mastery is the Art of Relaxation. You must make a conscientious effort to practice relaxing no matter how busy your day is. When you feel you don't have any time to relax, that is a sure sign to take five. If there is a situation that pushes you off center, you can choose to relax instead of react. Discovering what puts us in a blue funk gives us the opportunity to snap out of it. The relaxation response can become a way to lose the blues.

When you make the choice to stay calm at times when you could go wacko, you gain self-discipline and staying power. The more you relax, the more you develop the powerful presence of mind known as grace under pressure. As the yoga master Hariharananda states, "Calmness is Godliness."

Your secret formula is the power of Zen breathing. Use it to your advantage and get centered when stressful situations confront you. When you are stuck in gridlock or if a car cuts you off on the freeway, you can choose to remain cool and clearheaded. If your boss is going ballistic or you are forced to deal with rude people, choose to stay calm and centered. This approach is called going with the flow, and enables you to avoid wasting your energy and exhausting yourself. By staying cool you stay energized.

At the end of a difficult day, a great way to relax and recharge is to assume the Sponge Pose. Simply lie flat on the ground for up to five minutes. Listen to the spontaneous flow of your breath. Let yourself sink and melt into the floor, breathing slowly and steadily. On each Long Breath Out, mentally repeat the number "one" and feel your body become one with the magnetic core of Mother Earth. This simple relaxation technique also promotes Ch'i circulation, revitalizing you from head to toe.

As you can see, there are many opportunities throughout the day for you to Live Your Practice. I have touched on just a few. I'm sure you will discover many more. But please remember this: keep it Dr. Seuss simple. Do not think or try too hard. This interferes with your progress and causes your mind to spin. Don't fuss with it. It will come. Like a Samurai Cowgirl, when I fall off my horse, I get right back on. Just lighten up and go with the flow. There is always room to grow. Let Mental Fitness be your wakeup call. As Ralph Waldo Emerson once said, "Do the thing and you will have the power."

*Power comes by discipline
and by discipline alone.*

E. Stanley Jones

*Simply imagine it so,
then go about to prove it.*

Albert Einstein

THE SUPREME DISCIPLINE FORMULA

Be Patient. Enjoy the moment to moment journey.

Be Persistent. No excuses. Do it anyway, rain or shine. Stick to it like corn on a cob.

Be Passionate. Live it. Breathe it. Do it with love.

HOME SWEET HOME

Three is the magical number. In *The Wizard of Oz*, Dorothy clicked her heels three times to go home, and so can we. Take three deep breaths. Follow your heart home on the Long Breath Out.

One for the mind—to clear.

Two for the body—to center.

Three for the spirit—to soar.

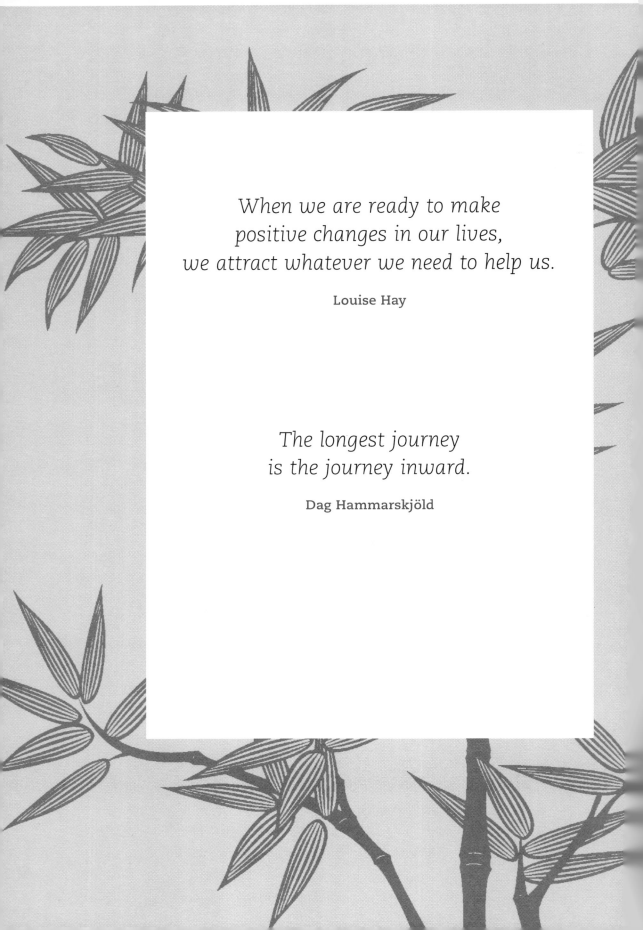

When we are ready to make
positive changes in our lives,
we attract whatever we need to help us.

Louise Hay

The longest journey
is the journey inward.

Dag Hammarskjöld

JOURNAL THE JOURNEY

Socrates said, "The unexamined life is not worth living." Journal writing is a tool we can use to explore the known and the unknown within ourselves. Examining our lives with pen and paper gives us a chance to listen compassionately to the voice of our hearts. Writing down our thoughts helps to clarify them. This provides an emotional cleansing and an honest time to get in touch with who we are. Be conscious of the fact that you are always learning and growing.

So, how do you do it? Get a blank notebook. Ask yourself, What is my purpose? What is my direction? What do I want to get out of this work? You will be recording the progress of your journey. There are no mistakes, only honest feedback. Don't censure or judge your feelings. Writing down the negatives helps you to look at them and remove them, one by one. The truth may be a bitter pill to swallow, but the truth can also set you free. Focusing on the positive creates a light that will always guide you through the darkness.

You have the choice to focus on your short or long term goals and chart your progress, or, you can go deeper and get in touch with your core essence. It is truly up to you.

Here are three powerful points to remember when journal writing and goal setting.

Visualization. Use your imagination to envision and create what you desire. Write down a clear description of your goal. Be specific. See and feel yourself achieving that goal. Act as if you are already there.

Affirmation. Make positive, personal statements about how you want to be and act. Always make them firmly and in the present tense.

Write them down, look at them often, and repeat them to yourself again and again, with feeling. Example: "I am one with my Divine nature and I have infinite, creative power."

Observation. Log your experiences every day. Write down the feelings you are having and the results you are getting. This daily feedback allows you to see your progress.

Here is a sample journal entry to get you started. Keep it simple and direct.

> *March 22*
> *Today, I practiced the Centered Breath around 7:30 a.m. It got easier. Breathing with my mouth closed still feels funny. To focus, I used a countdown of five to one on my exhalations. I did it for about five minutes. Emotional stuff came up from my past, but focusing on the breath flow helped to clear my head.*
> *Oh yeah, I'm still open to finding a purpose. My goal, right now, is just to make it through today more centered. More later.*

This wonderful process of journal writing is a form of mental workout. It requires your honest engagement and a commitment to follow through. Make it a ritual and do it with enthusiasm, which comes from the Greek words *en theos*, meaning "in God." Stay open to the possibilities that are yours for the asking and the receiving.

*Unless you turn around
and become as children,
you will by no means enter
the kingdom of heaven.*

Matthew 18:3

MY MESSAGE FOR INNER PEACE

I can tell you to live your practice and be mentally strong in the face of constant change and life's adversities. But I know this is easier said than done. Before I go, I'd like to share with you something permanent that can sustain you when everything seems impossible. Where do you find the power to follow through, no matter what?

You already possess it. Jesus said, "Behold, the Kingdom of God is within you." (Luke 17:21) The invisible source of power is unchanging, and resides in the center of your being. Some identify it as their higher self, soul, or spirit. What you choose to call it is up to you.

Turning within to this power and trusting in it gives you the inner strength to turn your dreams and visions into living reality. Having the faith of a child while planning like an adult will awaken this perfect power within you. Faith is the opposite of fear. Take a moment to breath in faith and breathe out fear—expelling doubts and distractions.

What has helped me to carry on when everything seemed unbearable is a little pearl of wisdom from Mahatma Gandhi: "Where love is, there God is also." This timeless expression reminds us to recognize and appreciate our spiritual connection to the source of all creation. God is love, our spiritual fuel.

As you journey down the road less traveled to inner peace, I look forward to seeing you along the way. The poem on the next page is a jewel of light to carry with you to nourish your soul and uplift your spirit.

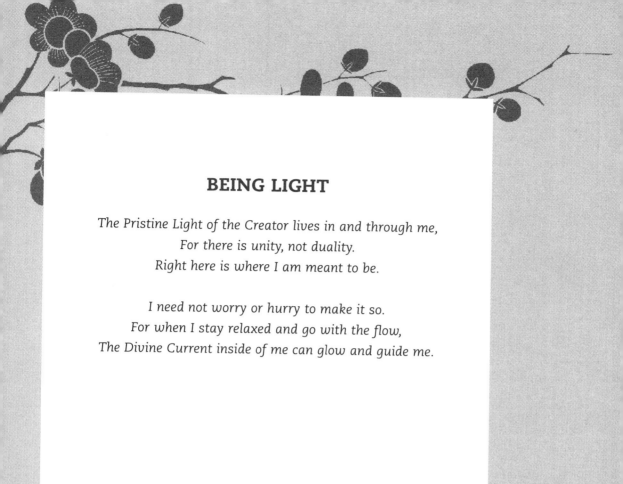

BEING LIGHT

The Pristine Light of the Creator lives in and through me,
For there is unity, not duality.
Right here is where I am meant to be.

I need not worry or hurry to make it so.
For when I stay relaxed and go with the flow,
The Divine Current inside of me can glow and guide me.

This is not

THE END

It is only the beginning.

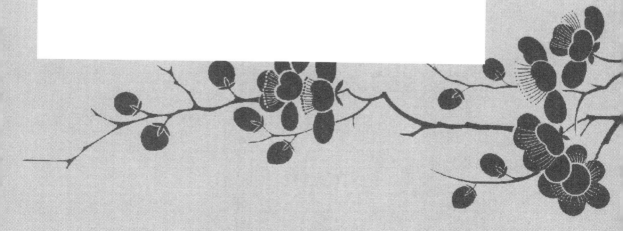

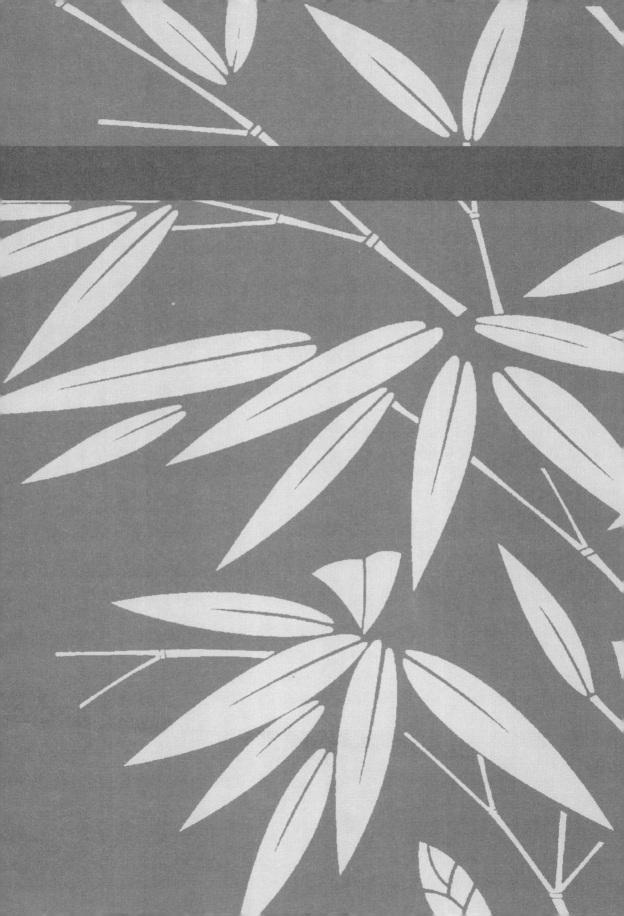

APPENDIXES

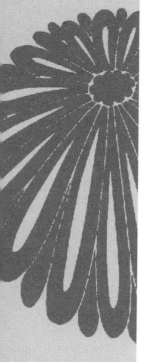

I am not discouraged,
because every wrong attempt discarded
is another step forward.

Thomas Edison

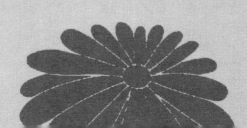

THE SEVEN LEVELS OF MENTAL FITNESS

The Foundation. It all begins here. The techniques in this book establish a base upon which we can build. A strong foundation gives us security, the ability to trust in ourselves, and confidence to stand our ground. First roots of love, then wings of freedom.

Self-Acceptance. Develop a positive and approving attitude toward yourself. Realize you are all right the way you are. With patience and self-love, you will achieve results easily and naturally.

Inner Power. As we progress in our practice, we develop self-respect, discipline, and a new sense of self-control. Building our strength from the inside out allows us to give ourselves orders, make decisions, and take action. We can snap to and do what must be done.

Compassion. To move forward we must remove the emotional obstacles that have hindered us. By releasing fear, jealousy, and anger, we can experience more love and compassion. Pure love continually forgives.

Honesty. We must learn to communicate effectively with ourselves and others. Honesty is always the best policy. Freedom is our gift when we speak the truth.

Inner Knowledge. As we mentally abstain from negativity, our positive qualities are given room to grow. Faith and intuition are strengthened. We have now moved from the stage of thinking to that of knowing.

Unity with Divinity. This is the highest level of Mental Fitness. By developing an attitude of gratitude, we become in tune with our spiritual nature. The invisible current flows through us and we are one with all of life.

KEYWORDS

Affirmation—A positive personal statement phrased in the present tense about the way you want to act, think, and be in your life.

Breath—Inspiration; spirit; air; animation.

Ch'i—Breath energy; electrical energy; a Chinese concept of mental and physical energy.

Ch'i Kung—Breath work; the soft internal art of disciplined breathing.

Compassion—To care with passion; the Latin root means "with love."

Concentration—To focus without distraction, either internally, or externally on an object or activity.

Control—to have charge of, direct, or pilot; but also to contain or reserve.

Discipline—to practice, exercising self-control; the ability to work systematically to achieve an objective; self-mastery.

Ego—the small, limited self; the conscious personality; self-importance.

Energy—power, current, force, heat; comes from the Greek word *ergon,* which means "work."

Fear—Anxiety, suspicion; a state of holding oneself back.

Flow—to proceed continuously; fluid, smooth; a peak performance state of clear-minded and effortless control.

Grace—Smooth and agile motion; dignity, honor; love in action, compassion, forgiveness, kindness.

Hara—Japanese term for the center of gravity and energy source in our lower abdomen, essential to both physical and mental balance; known in Chinese as the *t'an t'ien*.

Intuition—Direct inner knowing without intellectual reasoning; insight.

Meditation—to direct attention from the outer world to our inner world; relaxing and listening; a spiritual art.

Mindfulness—Attentiveness; present, centered awareness of what is happening in the moment-to-moment flow of life.

Soul—Inner self; spiritual being; animating principle or essence; courage.

Spirit—Breath of God; inspiration; the force animating living beings.

Visualization—The technique of using mental imagery to create what you want in your life. The mind thinks in pictures.

Wisdom—Understanding of what is true; clear thinking balanced with insight; experience.

Yin and Yang—Inseparable and complementary parts of a unified whole. Yin is passive and feminine, associated with Water and Earth; Yang is active and masculine, associated with Fire and Air.

Zazen—The practice of Zen; literally, "sitting meditation."

Zen—Inner discipline of the mind; objectless concentration; deep silence; meditation; from the Sanskrit word *dhyana* and the Chinese *ch'an*.

RECOMMENDED READING

This is not a comprehensive bibliography. Instead, it is a brief list of highly recommended books for interested readers to explore and consult. These books touch on many aspects of the material covered here, and have helped me tremendously in deepening my understanding of the fascinating subject of mind-body communication.

Benson, Herbert. *The Relaxation Response*. New York: Avon, 1975.

Boerstler, Richard, and Hulen Kornfeld. *Life to Death: Harmonizing the Transition*. Vermont: Healing Arts Press, 1995.

Chopra, Deepak. *Ageless Body, Timeless Mind*. New York: Harmony Books, 1993.

Deshimaru, Taisen. *The Zen Way to the Martial Arts*. New York: Penguin Books, 1982.

Dürckheim, Karlfried Graf von. *Hara: The Vital Centre Of Man*. London: HarperCollins, 1962.

Gawain, Shakti. *Creative Visualization*. New York: MJF Books, 1978.

Hanh, Thich Nhat. *The Miracle Of Mindfulness*. Boston: Beacon Press, 1975.

Hay, Louise. *Heart Thoughts*. Carson, California: Hay House, 1990.

Huang, Chungliang Al, and Jerry Lynch. *Thinking Body, Dancing Mind*. New York: Bantam Books, 1992.

Jeffers, Susan. *End the Struggle and Dance with Life*. New York: St. Martin's Press, 1996.

Maltz, Maxwell. *Psycho-Cybernetics.* New York: Pocket Books, 1960.

Norris, Chuck. *The Secret Power Within: Zen Solutions to Real Problems.* Canada: Little Brown & Co., 1996.

Sokei-an. Farkas, Mary, ed. *The Zen Eye.* New York: Weatherhill, 1993.

Zi, Nancy. *The Art of Breathing.* New York: Bantam Books, 1986.

ACKNOWLEDGMENTS

Over the years, I have learned from many individuals who have helped guide me and support my vision. I would like to take this opportunity to thank them.

Jehovah. God inside me. The Father of Truth and The Mother of Love—All my thanks for this gift and the ability to share Your Light.

Mommy, Maruko. Daddy, Jim. My two beautiful sisters, Yuriko and Fumiko—I love you beyond words.

James Wing Woo—My ultimate Sifu. Thank you for supporting my vision of mind, body, and soul unity. Your supreme patience and genius eye for good and bad has made my teaching possible.

Dr. Richard Boerstler— Thank you for your continual support and love, and for reminding me that the Way will show the Way.

Joshu Sasaki Roshi and Leonard Cohen—Thank you beyond words for your true love.

David Noble and the staff of Weatherhill—Thank you for refining the text and giving the book a beautiful Zenlike form.

To all my students—Thank you for supporting the work. I love you all.

Ronnie—You caught me in mid-air and brought me down gently to the ground. Thank you for Roots of Love and Wings of Freedom. I love you.

A special thanks to: June (Sugar) Brown, Bill Braunstein, Marie Chase, Mary Farkas, Ralph Hadsell, Dion Jackson, Carmalita Maracci, Gene Marinaccio, Joe Sample, Pat Strong, Marie Sutor, and Johanon Vigoda.

To all of those not mentioned, in the interest of brevity: please accept my heartfelt gratitude. Ti amo.

ABOUT THE AUTHOR

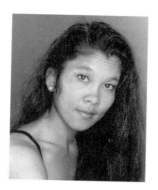

MICHIKO J. ROLEK is the great-grandaughter of Sokei-an Sasaki, the first Zen master to make his home in America. This unique heritage has been a deep influence on her life and helped set her on the path of spiritual awakening. She shares her own Christian Zen philosophy through her teaching and writing.

Formerly a jewelry designer and a professional dancer, Michiko now teaches her own unique system of mind/body fitness, a synthesis of twenty years of intensive study and practice of the martial arts, yoga, and dance. While working extensively as a Mental and Inner Fitness coach, she continues to fine tune her mind-body communication skills.

The "weathermark" identifies this book as a production of Weatherhill, Inc., publishers of fine books on Asia and the Pacific. Editorial supervision, book and cover design: D.S. Noble. Production supervision: Bill Rose. Printing and binding: Daamen, Inc. The typeface used is PMN Cæcelia.